T0105373

Fifty Shades
of
Pleasure

Fifty Shades of Pleasure

A BEDSIDE COMPANION

Sex Secrets that Hurt So Good

MARISA BENNETT

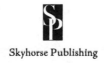

Skyhorse Publishing

Skyhorse Publishing books may be purchased in bulk at special discounts for sales promotion, corporate gifts, fund-raising, or educational purposes. Special editions can also be created to specifications. For details, contact the Special Sales Department, Skyhorse Publishing, 307 West 36th Street, 11th Floor, New York, NY 10018 or info@skyhorsepublishing.com.

Skyhorse® and Skyhorse Publishing® are registered trademarks of Skyhorse Publishing, Inc.®, a Delaware corporation.

Visit our website at www.skyhorsepublishing.com.

10 9 8 7 6 5 4 3

Library of Congress Cataloging-in-Publication Data is available on file.

ISBN: 978-1-62087-334-2

Printed in the United States of America

DEDICATION

To Monica and Becky, who taught
me how to be myself.

CONTENTS

INTRODUCTION

U nless you've been living under a rock re-
cently, you've noticed that new erotica
novels have pounced on pop-culture,
teased it, tempted it, and left it begging for more.
Over the past few years, e-books allowed some liter-
ary smut enthusiasts to sneakily read their erotica in
public spaces, but reading sexy lit was still a little
taboo. Now and for the first time, men and wom-
en—from yoga moms to twenty-somethings—are
unabashedly knocking down store clerks to get their
hands on hardcore hardcovers.

I wanted to write a book that embraced the
naughtier sides of sex, empowered men and women
to be bold with their sexuality, and of course, that
cheered on the proud erotica reader. While parts of
this book highlight what you might call, "vanilla
sex," much of the content focuses on BDSM, an ac-
ronym that condenses bondage & discipline, dominance & submission, and sadism & masochism. This
quaint set of letters umbrellas a whole host of dirty
little sex tricks and lifestyles. This book is meant
to focus on some of the spiciest sides of BDSM and
erotic play that will allow you and your partner to
take the reins of your sexy time—and maybe smack
it in the ass a little. I hope you enjoy.

ABOUT THE AUTHOR

Marisa Bennett graduated from the University of Massachusetts Amherst with a degree in English Literature, and she has a definite kinky side! Her hard limits are ice cream with nuts and skydiving. She lives with her husband in Minnesota.

Chapter One

Mind-Blowing Sex Techniques

"A loving pair become blind with passion in the heat of congress, and go on with great impetuosity, paying not the least regard to excess."

—Vātsyāyana
Kama Sutra

"I could play the woman
with mine eyes,
And braggart with
my tongue!"

—Shakespeare
Macbeth

You can't get to kinky sex without some kinky instructions. Sometimes trying something new (or trying something old with a new approach) can be difficult when all you have to go on is personal experience, or a partner who doesn't always verbalize what he or she wants. These introductory tips—from performing oral sex that will leave you both gasping for more, to acrobatic sex positions—are part of the artillery you'll need for your sex-time stockpile. So get out your notepad and ace your next anatomy exam!

ORAL SEX TECHNIQUES FOR HER:
Performing Knee-Quakingly Great Fellatio

THE MOVE

It's no secret that men love blowjobs. Unfortunately, giving sensational fellatio isn't a gift that just drops down on us from the heavens; you have to know the choreography. Grasping everything—from the basics, to the naughty little things your guy won't ask for (but wants)—will be the difference in whether he just loves blowjobs, or he loves *your* blowjobs.

MAKING IT HAPPEN

First and foremost, "a blow job's a blow job's a blow job," is not an effective mantra. Whether you give him head spontaneously, or prefer to stick with the week you have your period, you still need to approach it as if there's nothing you'd rather be doing for him. Unenthusiastic fellatio feels the same way to him as unenthusiastic cunnilingus does to you—it's a waste of time and a little bit irritating. So make this an experience that will have him breathless in between each holler of your name.

Starting him off:

Begin by teasing him: Sensually nibble at his ears, and kiss him down his neck and chest, and down along his beltline. When you undo his pants, do this slowly, and make sure not to go straight for the goods; it's always best to make him work up an appetite. When you have him at your mercy, feel free to tease him for a little while, even kissing and licking from sensitive areas like his knees, trailing up his inner thighs and right to the inside of his hips. Start by taking his shaft in your hand and licking his balls—if you can take his balls in your mouth, even better. Use your tongue to massage as you go.

Getting his blood pumping:

If you're going to remember anything, remember to keep his penis lubricated. When you take his penis in your mouth, use your saliva to get his whole shaft wet. And don't worry—not being able to "deep throat" will not prevent you from giving him phenomenal head. With the help of your saliva, use your hand as an extension of your mouth as you go up and down his shaft. Keep your grip firm, but there's no need to squeeze him to death. Everyone is different, so feel free to take moments to be verbal and ask how firm he wants your grip to be, and how fast or slowly to go. Remember to keep massaging his penis with a lubricated hand while you ask questions—this is also a good way for you to take a breather if you're getting tired, without letting him lose steam.

Try rotating your hand in a circular motion as you go up and down his shaft, being sure to massage on and around the tip on your way up. If you're a good multi-tasker, massage his balls with your free hand. Take things further by using your saliva or a lubricant, and continue the blow job while massaging his balls with one or two hands—even pulling on his sack a little (but not too hard). Your saliva on his balls will make it feel like your mouth is on his penis and his sack at the same time. When you're in the area, also try massaging his perineum, which is the space between his scrotum and his anus. This area is super sensitive, and will produce a reaction somewhere in between moaning your name in surprise, and pulling your hair from brimming rapture.

The kinky extra step that will blow his mind:

This addition depends entirely on your personal comfort level and that of your partner. Experiment by stroking his perineum and inserting your (lubricated) finger into his anus near or during his climax for a prostate massage. Massaging this area can cause men to come even without genital stimulation, so if you're already giving him head, his orgasm will be absolutely explosive. When your finger is inside him, move it towards his front in a slight "come hither" motion, going slowly and varying the pressure. Continuing this through his climax will have him erupting in ecstasy and gasping for air.

The finish line:

How you finish him off is almost as important as how you get there. Most importantly, don't treat his semen like it's radioactive. If you can have his penis in your mouth, you can handle touching a little fluid;

"No pleasure endures
unseasoned by
variety."

—Publius Syrus

otherwise, you're just insulting him. If you choose to swallow—hooray! You're probably helping to prevent breast cancer! (Studies have shown that women who swallow a couple of tablespoons of semen a few times a week have lower occurrences of breast cancer, though your risk will not increase if you don't swallow.) If you are wary of those pesky gag reflexes and would prefer not to swallow, there are options. You can finish him using your hands, or even suggest that he comes on your chest. Lubricate his penis with your mouth, and then have him put his shaft in between your breasts while he goes over the edge. This is a kinky way to finish him off that will have him fantasizing about the image later on.

Oral Sex Techniques for Him: *Performing Earth-Shatteringly Great Cunnilingus*

THE MOVE

Bumping uglies is great, but sometimes you need a little something special—a little extra care and attention. Of course, I mean cunnilingus. If you're going to be tying each other up (more on that later!), you want to make sure he knows what to do when he heads south. Here are a few tips to help him out!

MAKING IT HAPPEN

Enthusiasm is important here, for you and him, just as it was with the blow job. It's also important to communicate, since everybody's got his or her own preferences (different strokes for different vaginas, as I always say). Have him start slow, with plenty of kisses down your stomach and on the inside of your thighs. Once you're warmed up and ready, he can start teasing your clitoris. He can start by making slow, lazy circles around your clitoris, or have him use his tongue to write letters across your sexy bits. Have him change it up, moving his tongue in varying patterns and at different speeds. Try having him suck gently on your clitoris and rub it gently across his teeth.

His hands should be busy touching, stroking, and caressing you, paying special attention to the places he knows you like to be touched. He can also use his fingers, especially when he takes breaks to kiss you or pay extra attention to your boobs. He can do this by rubbing your clitoris, or filling you with a finger or two. As he goes, encourage him to go deeply and stimulate your G-spot. To find it, he should insert one or two fingers gently into you, and then slowly move it in a "come hither" wiggle, stroking you inside, right by your bellybutton. If he can pat his head and rub his stomach at the same time, he can probably go down and finger you at the same time. Stellar tongue action and dedicated hands can send you over the edge! Have him do this as your budding climax creeps up on you (pulling his hair, increased moaning, or shouts of "I'm going to come!" will tell him it's time). Right as you're coming to a peak, having him suck lightly on your clitoris will have you red, hot, and screaming his name.

WILD SEX POSITION:
The Desktop Duo

THE MOVE

After a long day at work, there's nothing better to help you unwind than a vigorous, stress-releasing romp with your partner. When this happy hour special just can't wait, make him sweep the clutter off his desk and get down to serious business. Try out these hot sex moves on his desk, and be his after work delight!

MAKING IT HAPPEN

His desk is the best work space, especially when he's working hard for you. While he's sitting at his desk, sensually straddle a leg over his lap and seat yourself on the desk's edge right in front of him. Spice this first step up by doing some of the work for him and keep the clothing to a minimum, whether you wear a cute nightie with no underwear, or just don one of his work shirts with sexy lingerie underneath.

Tighten Your Schedule:

If he hasn't shot up from his chair already, sexily bring one leg over his shoulder and urge him towards you to a standing position. With your leg still draped over his shoulder and the other tip-toeing the floor, keep your bum leaned on the desk for support. Having him enter you from this angle will be sure to give him a super-tight fit that will move his attention from a hard day's work to . . . just being hard.

Cross-Referencing:

Switch up the position you're already in by moving yourself slightly back onto his desk and lying down. As he continues to stand, criss-cross your legs, putting your right foot on his right shoulder, and your left foot on his left shoulder. The higher up your legs are crossed above the knee, the tighter you'll feel to him. Have him hold on to your hips or thighs for

"One half of the
world cannot understand
the pleasures
of the other."
—Jane Austen
Emma

support while you clutch the desk. Feel free to move your feet from his shoulders and pivot your hips to the side, keeping your torso straight. This take on the criss-crossing move will have him feeling you from a whole new angle.

Doing the Dirty Work:

Success in the workplace really shows when you give it your all. Lie down the length of his desk, wrapping your legs around him as he kneels on top of the desk in front of you. Scoot yourself forward so that your ass rests on his thighs and he can enter you with ease. You can keep your legs around his waist or have them straight up in the air where he can clutch them for support. The elevation of your hips will get him so deep in, he'll forget about all the paperwork he just threw to the floor.

WILD SEX POSITION:
The Whirlpool

THE MOVE

Adding water to your repertoire is the fastest way to steam things up between you and your partner. The skinny-dip tryst skips the hassle of undressing and goes straight for the slippery samba. For the Jacuzzi enthusiast, or the claw-foot tub aficionado, here are some techniques to use to get the waves rolling.

MAKING IT HAPPEN

Getting dirty while you soap each other up can be a spontaneous rendezvous as you both get ready for work, or a sensually crafted spa-like getaway with candles and incense. Whichever you choose, slide into these sexy positions the next time you've got your partner cornered with a little H_2O.

The Classic:

If you're the type who likes to get slammed against a wall, the shower is a perfect place to do it. The combination of hot water pouring down on you and your partner, and the immediate, sexy visual of one another stripped down and covered in slippery suds is enough to get even the most frigid all hot and bothered. When he pins you against the tile wall—and he will—sneak a little nearby conditioner and start massaging his shaft and his balls. This spa treatment will have him ready for anything. Raise a leg to his hips so that he knows you want to be wrapped tightly around him, then have him pick you up by the hips, and let the shower wall support you as he thrusts into you. If he has a hard time keeping you up, or you find you're having a hard time participating, keep one leg wrapped around him and support your other foot with the corner of the shower or the edge of the bathtub.

The Double-Header:

Removable shower heads are the gods'—or Home Depot's—gift to sex. Get those hard to reach areas by facing the shower wall with your arms up and hands palming the tile. Having him stand behind you will give him free reign to rub you down, kiss your neck, and aim that shower head where he thinks you've been a naughty girl. Let him enter you from behind, and if you're lucky enough to have two faucets, the primary faucet can spray water where he's thrusting you into ecstasy, while he lets the second showerhead pound its way to your climax.

Bubbling Over:

There's a reason why flexibility and sex go hand-in-hand. This position is easier for the guy (in other words, he just shows up), and requires a little bend-ability from the girl. As he stands under the hot stream of water, have him enter you from behind as you slowly bend over. Being able to touch your hands to the shower floor will get him twenty-thousand leagues into you, which will give your G-spot extra attention. When he has a rapid pace going, his balls will rhythmically slap against your clitoris, giving you double the stimulation. If you feel like he's riding the tide faster than you, move your hands from the floor to the edge of the tub. This change of angle will bring you into shallow waters, slowing down the pace a little and let you concentrate on your own aquatic pleasure.

The Tub Tantra:

With the shower running and a few inches of water to keep you warm, lie down the length of the bathtub. Encourage him to give you a good, soapy rubdown before you begin, so that you can slide back and forth in the tub more easily. Have him kneel down in the tub in front of you, lifting one of your legs up in the air, holding onto it as he moves into you and straddles the other. Rest your leg on his shoulder and have him use your thigh to pull himself deeper in and out of you. The sideways angle of your pelvis against him will fill you up, give you a sultry sensation that missionary style alone can't provide, and offer your clitoris that extra attention for the build-up you need.

The Typhoon Twist:

This next position gets you tied up, twisted and extra close up with your partner. Sit down in a filled bathtub or on the bench of a Jacuzzi facing your partner. Straddle your partner with both of your legs wrapped around one another in a tight, tantalizing embrace. Both of you should be sitting up so that your soapy, wet chests can silkily rub against one another, letting your passion boil over with a seriously seductive make-out session. To get even closer, lock your arms with his from under each of your knees, which will help your balance. If this position gets too tricky, have him lean back against the wall of the tub, and with the help of his shoulders or the bathtub's edge, you can continue to ride him from on top while looking like a sexy siren.

WILD SEX POSITION:
Full Throttle

THE MOVE

Don't subdue your sexual energy just because you're outside of the house. Cars come in all shapes and sizes, and lucky for you, so do sex positions. Reclining seats, well-timed music, moon roofs, and soft leather are sexy ingredients for a very tasty tryst. When you can't keep your hands off of each other long enough to make it home, pull over and test out the bells and whistles your car dealer never told you about.

MAKING IT HAPPEN

Sex in a car will get your engine roaring in a way that being in a bedroom just can't—the close quarters and fear of getting caught will have your windows fogging up in no time.

Power Steering:

Sometimes guys just want you to take the wheel. When he's in the driver's seat, get him revved up by leaning over and kissing his neck and nipping at his ears, unbuttoning his shirt as you go. Gently run your hands along his skin until he's tingling with excitement. When his engine's humming, move over to the driver's seat with your hands on the wheel. Face the windshield, and slowly slide down on his shaft. Use the steering wheel for support as you ride him, giving all of your horse-power to this sexy take on reverse-cowgirl.

Backseat Booty:

If the front seat has you feeling cramped, move to the backseat where those thoughtful automobile manufacturers have conveniently supplied you with a couch. Have him sit in the middle seat, where you can easily straddle him. This position gives him a full view and great access to your body, where he can hold you tightly as you drive him into oblivion. This position will let him go nice and deep, and since his back is supported by the car's seat, your clitoris will grind right up against him as you go. With his hands on your hips, try arching your back as far back as possible, using either his shoulders or the back of the seat for support, so that the tip of his penis rubs against the inside wall of your vagina. If the windows are rolled up, you'll be sure to work up a steamy sweat, which will make the ride nice and slick. Be sure to roll the windows down when you're done to get a refreshing breeze while you cool down.

Driving Stick:

The open road is full of possibilities—and so is road head. Of course, your partner probably has a hard enough time concentrating on the road if you're kissing his neck, so giving him head will be sure to send you into oncoming traffic. It's better to try this when the engine isn't running, where he'll be able to lean his head back and be glad you decided to take his car. Giving him head while you're in the passenger's seat is a tricky move—your mouth is perpendicular to where it normally is, which will make his penis feel like it doesn't fit the way it should. To avoid accidentally biting him, either be hyperaware of how your mouth fits and go slowly, or move your knees to the ground of the passenger's seat so you're closer to a typical blowjob position. He'll be able to use the steering wheel—or your ponytail—to grip when you're sending him over the edge.

DIRTY TALK DOS AND DON'TS

Talking dirty is one of the hottest ways to build sexual chemistry with your partner and invigorate your tumble in the sack, but it's oddly one of the basics that couples fear the most. Here are the yeas and nays to guide you through sexplicit scripts in bed.

Dos

Do get confident. No one expects you to become a linguistic porn star overnight, but self-deprecation and uncomfortable wriggling as

"Be still when you have
nothing to say; when
genuine passion
moves you,
say what you've got
to say, and
say it hot."

—D. H. Lawrence

you spit the naughty verbiage will not only ring hollow, it'll be sure to kill the mood.

Do be honest. The simplest way to start talking dirty is by asking for what you want or acknowledging what you like. Complimenting the person is a two-way turn-on, and it's okay to start off innocently. Saying, "I love how you look on top of me," or "you feel amazing inside me," certainly won't crown you for your verbal filth, but it'll get the conversation rolling.

Do be descriptive. Whether it's via text or face-to-face, tell your partner what you want to do, and equally importantly, what you want to be done to you. If you're not ready for total vulgarity, use sensual words and lingering descriptions as you speak. The more descriptive the imagery, the closer you and your partner will be to actually feeling it.

Do break your comfort zone. The reason dirty talk is so sexy is because most people don't regularly shout from the rooftops that they want to fuck the shit out of their partners. Reserving naughty talk for the bedroom or whispering it so others can't hear makes you the someone who can be brought home to mom, and then later completely ravished. Say things you wouldn't normally say, be direct, and avoid childish terms like, "thing," "her," and "down there."

Do swear to God. Particularly if you don't cuss like a construction worker in normal conversation, swearing in bed shows primal, unabridged lust for your partner. Feel free to swear in most any form, whether it's used as a verb ("Oh my God, FUCK me"), a superlative ("You have the fucking sexiest dick"), an adjective ("Holy shit, I want to be inside your wet fucking pussy"), or your average exclamation whilst moaning or mid-climax ("OHH, FUCK!"). Swear away!

Don'ts

Don't be wrong. If anything you say has the potential to make your partner laugh in your face, or is just plain ridiculous, don't say it.

Telling your lover that you have the biggest cock she's ever seen—or that you're going to give him the best he's ever had—could very well be completely false. If it is true, then your partner can tell you.

Don't say your ex's name. This is Relationship 101, let alone Dirty Talk 101. Saying your lover's name will be sure to make him or her super hot, but saying the wrong name is the fastest way to get a bedside object thrown at you or a door slammed in your face.

Don't be too literal. Telling your girl, "I'm going to make your eyes roll back in your head" may be totally true, but imagery that could also be confused with an epileptic seizure is not going to get her there. Focus on things you want him or her to feel, and less on what may literally happen.

Don't be the wrong kind of dirty. A filthy mouth can get your partner all sorts of riled up, but saying, "I'm going to shit on your chest," isn't the kind of vulgarity you're looking for.

Don't use baby talk or genital pet names. While baby talk might be cutesy during a snuggle sesh, it has no place in the sack. Similarly, calling your man's penis your "little soldier," or the like, will have that GI shrinking back into his barracks. Having names for your own genitalia is a close cousin. Calling your penis "The Crusader" or "Thunder God," or calling your vagina "The Pink Palace" during sex is just asking to be told otherwise. Stick with the dirty classics like "cock," "dick," and "pussy," with various blood-pumping adjectives attached.

Chapter 2

Spank Me, Baby!

"Pain is no evil,
Unless it
conquers us."

—Charles Kingsley

"Sweet is pleasure
after pain."

—John Dryden
Alexander's Feast

INTRO:
The Hows and Whys of Spanking

Before there were sex playrooms, before there were dildos, and before there were floggers, even, there was an open palm. Spanking is the very first step into the painfully hot side of your sexy rendezvous, with a little something for everyone. While there's no question why the sweet sides of sex keep hot-blooded bodies coming back for more, it's harder to imagine why a good wallop would have the same effect. As it turns out, your body releases chemicals, like endorphins and adrenaline, when triggered by strenuous activity, stimulation, and even pain—a trifecta that is abundant during sex. So when your partner's brimming lust gets hand-delivered, the combination of your arousal and a little surge of pain can bring your romp, and eventual climax, to a whole new level. Beginning with baby steps (or maybe baby spanks!) this chapter will show you the A-Zs of one of the most exciting and simple additions to your sexual repertoire.

THE BAREHANDED BENCHMARK

THE MOVE

If you have never felt the tingle of a freshly spanked rump, it's best to start with the basics. No, not the flogger; we'll get there. First, start with what you were born with: your bare hands. Whether you want to be the spanker or the spankee, barehanded spanking is a way to tap into a lusty—even primal—side of sex. It can also be an amazing way to connect with your partner mid-romp. While spanking can involve games of power play, in the throes of sex spanking is more often than not, a reaction—as our team of scientists like to call it, the "OMG, you feel amazing, I just have to grab or hit something!" response. Whichever your fancy, doing it barehanded will inspire a new side of your sex life that is stingingly sweet. So warm up those palms or scoot up your bum, and let the spanking begin!

MAKING IT HAPPEN

With the beginning stages of spanking, you have to test the waters before you jump in. As the spanker, if you're unsure if your partner wants to try spanking

FIFTY SHADES OF PLEASURE

with you, and you fear, "The Talk," try warming up with it the next time she's on top. Caress or massage her ass a little, and when you're feeling particularly enthralled, give her a swift—but not too swift—smack to the bum. Body language (or her screaming your name) should indicate whether you have the green light or a halting red stop sign.

Once you have the go ahead, treat spanking like candy. If you have too little, you might be missing out on something sweet. If you have too much, you've spoiled an appetite and you might never be allowed back in the candy store again. Incorporate palm-to-cheek meetings when things are particularly fiery to send both of your sexual trajectories soaring. Feel free to spank multiple times in a row with a slow, firm rhythm, either open-palmed or with your palm slightly cupped. This can occur with the spankee on top ("The Reach Around," if you will), or doggie-style, where you'll have a better view of the bright red handprint you'll be making on your partner's tush.

The subtle nuances of asking to be spanked aren't much different than asking to spank. If you and your partner have good sexual chemistry, chances are that the risk of asking is worth the reward. Declaring, "I want you to spank me," while out to dinner with the in-laws may not be the right time to mention it, but kissing your partner's neck and whispering it in

34

"No empty handed
man can lure
a bird."

—Geoffrey Chaucer
The Canterbury Tales

his ear while you're on top of him in bed just might. If you're uncomfortable with asking directly, move your partner's hands to your hips during sex, and slowly bring them to cup or squeeze your ass. Go so far as to take your partner's hands and do the smacking yourself. At that point, he or she should be able to infer that you're saying, "Spank Me, Baby!"

Propping It Up

THE MOVE

After you and your partner have covered the basics of barehanded, it's time to use a prop. Using a prop while spanking will increase your ability to deliver a good thump, or intensify a spanking that you're about to receive. With every good thwap to the ass you enjoy, more blood flows to the very sensitive nerve endings in the cheeks, which also means more blood flow and impact are sent to the very sensitive nerve endings located right next door. Incorporating props is an exciting way to liven up your sex life, not just because it's something new, but also because it involves forethought. While spontaneous sex is nothing to scoff at, there's something undeniably sexy about knowing your partner thinks about doing you so often that he or she went out and bought a toy.

MAKING IT HAPPEN

The props you and your partner use don't necessarily need to have blockbuster production value. You can use household items like the time-honored classics, the hairbrush and the ping-pong paddle. Both of these items are easily wielded, and while they'll certainly pack some punch, the spankee won't necessarily fear sitting down for the next week. A ping-pong paddle is usually encased in a thin layer of leather or rubber, which will end each blow with a slick smack. A hairbrush is more multifaceted. The flat end of the brush will deliver much the same impact as the paddle, while the bristled end (either hair or plastic with soft nubs) will add a prickly sensation to switch up the feel of each cheeky encounter.

If you're looking for an excuse to buy your props, there are paddles available that will bring your spanking session anywhere from sweetly sensual all the way to nastily naughty. For the former effect, try using a fur-lined paddle. The fuzzy addition to a firm paddle softens the sting of spanking, and can also be used to massage, caress, and seduce the spankee throughout its use. If you'd prefer something with ten times the zing, studded paddles are the take-no-prisoners approach to dishing out a good thumping. The studs create further pressure points to spike up the sexy mix of pleasure and pain. With these tools under your belt (you can use that, too!), your armory of sexilicious spankers is well on its way!

Teach Me a Lesson

THE MOVE

An armory of spanking techniques must be accompanied by a bit of role-playing. Whether you're dressing up as a leather-clad dominatrix, a sexy cop, a dirty doctor, or a naughty [insert profession here], role-playing gives an adrenaline shot to your sexcapades. The key to these games, of course, is doing the things you wouldn't do in everyday life, particularly if it has a pinch of spice and feels a little bit wrong. Sure, you might not normally go hiking, but role-playing as two adoring lovers in a mountainside field of lilacs isn't what you're looking for to sexify your lust sessions (unless it involves ropes and carabiners). So be the bad girl or the naughty boy and go for the Oscar in your next performance.

MAKING IT HAPPEN

For simplicity's sake, let's pretend you and your partner want to live out the Naughty Schoolgirl fantasy. It may sound overdone, but there's a reason why Britney Spears's "Baby One More Time" was so damn successful: It's hot. Not only is it super sexy, but it's a low-maintenance and low-cost way to get your and your partner's blood pumping.

First, pick out the wardrobe. Shopping online for schoolgirl skirts is a sure thing; otherwise, try second-hand, or of course, your local naughty gift shop. Once you have your costume, you're nearly ready for that after school special. Pair the skirt with whichever tightly fitting button-up blouse, T-shirt, or cardigan you already own, a pair of knee socks, and high heels—preferably Mary Janes, if you have them. Add some pigtails or French braids, and you've got one sexy schoolgirl on your hands.

Staying in character is one of the more important challenges of role-playing. Saying, "this is stupid," and "I feel silly," with stiff body language is the fastest way to get a big fat F on your exam. Confidence is sexy, so take control of your end of the bargain, whether it's the naughty schoolgirl or the professor she's staying after class with. Use your Dirty Talk Do's to get the scene playing out: Bite your lip as you tell your "professor" how badly you need to practice for your oral exams, or give your schoolgirl some corporal punishment for not handing in her homework on time. Making varsity never felt so good!

No schoolgirl scenario—or role-playing scenario, for that matter—would be complete without a nice dose of spanking. The point is to be bad, so get your palms, ruler, or clipboard out to give some serious detention. Bend your schoolgirl over your knee to punish her for being too cheeky, asking her to count as you spank and call you sir. Schoolgirl skirts are short for a reason, so make good use of them! Pull her skirt up and use your thick dictionary to remind her why she's staying after class. Those pigtails aren't just for show, either. Whether you're the one pulling her hair or getting your hair pulled, a little animalistic aggression will get you everywhere in your dirty scene. Pigtails are a perfect hairdo for a from-behind ride, so pull her by the reins and slap her ass to get her really going.

Step up your sexy performance: Buy additional props for spanking and branch out to different roles, even if it means that she's the whistling construction worker and he's the innocent passerby. Have fun with your wicked side and break the rules!

"Would you do me
the great kindness,
Madame,
of allowing me to bite
and pinch your
lovely flesh while
I'm at my fuckery?"

—Marquis de Sade
Philosophy in the Bedroom

℃

FLOG ME GENTLY

THE MOVE

Flogging takes prop-use to the next level (or five). A typical flogger is a spanking device that has a handle (otherwise known as a "pommel") with flowing tails attached, generally of the same length. These tails can be made up of leather, rubber, plastic, rope, horse hair, chain, or other fabrics, and can be used in a variety of ways throughout your mischievous spanking session. Floggers can be used to discipline your naughty partner, or to push your limits further than you ever thought you could go, and then some. This kind of erotic play is the ultimate destination for endorphin junkies. The more pain you take from your partner's flogger, the more you gain from that sweet release. From punishment and dominance play to flogging on a whim, this method of nasty pleasure makes even Cat Woman purr.

MAKING IT HAPPEN

The flogger is most often used for "discipline" purposes, where the spankee lies face down or leans over a chair, table, pillow, or even your very own spanking bench. The flogger can be administered with rapid flicks, which will bite steadily at the skin to get you and your partner hollering with excitement. For more sting to your swing, use a harder, slower pace, which will deliver a serious smack, as well as heighten anticipation between each impact. Before, after, or in between, lightly drag the tails of the flogger along your partner's ass or future flog-zone to tickle and taunt. This will provide relief in between blows, as well as get your partner all tingly with goose bumps for the next round.

Knowing which regions to target is extremely important. Generally speaking, the areas that scream "flog me!" are the back of the thighs, the shoulders, and of course, that booty. Unless you and your partner think a stint in the emergency room or a jail cell is super hot, it is important to stay away from the head, face, neck, spine, and soft tissue like the stomach, where all those important organs hang out. Flogging can be ultra sexy, but it's important to use your toys safely!

Pardon the yuck, but keep your flogger clean! Flogging isn't for the faint of...well, the faint . . . so if your sessions are especially intense, be prepared for welts and even broken skin or bleeding. Never use an unwashed flogger for multiple partners, and when you do clean it after each use, use disinfectants like antibacterial soap, leather cleaner, and bleach, depending on the material of the flogger. When you have these bases covered, flog it out of the park!

THE POST-SPANKING POSTERIOR

THE MOVE

With every good spanking, there needs to be equally good aftercare. Spanking play is to test your physical limits and invigorate your sexuality, to find new ways to bond with your partner, and naturally, to arouse. The best spanking rendezvous shouldn't leave you or your partner trembling in a corner after you've finished. If you are setting out for a no-holds-barred approach to spanking and BDSM play, then the post-spanking massage is a must-do to come down from a painfully good spanking summit and soothe those rosy cheeks.

MAKING IT HAPPEN

There's no doubt about it—spanking is an ass kicking. Whether the red-hot mark left on you or your partner's glutes is in the shape of a hand that meant business, the tip of a riding crop, or reads the word

"SLUT" from a particularly naughty paddle you purchased, they're going to need some attention. Lay the spankee down on the bed, your lap, or another soft surface, and lightly caress along the back, then the thighs, and then slowly begin to massage the bare bum. If you still feel like role-playing, tell the spankee he or she has done a good job and deserves the massage being given—anything negative is a Dirty Talk Don't. Rub massage oils or calming creams on areas that were given the most attention during the spanking. If you suspect there will be bruising (or can already see it), the massage will reduce soreness and increase circulation. Aftercare isn't just about the physical strain of spanking, it's also emotionally important. If your spanking exploits are particularly rough, the spankee may need a little extra affection and reminders of self-worth. Any games of power play and possibly degradation need to be cut as soon you've finished so there is no emotional confusion.

When choosing massage oils and creams, it is important to know what you're looking for. If you want to go all natural, essential oils like eucalyptus will be a wakeup for the skin, whereas jasmine and lavender will be more calming. If purchased in pure form, these oils *need* to be diluted with other base oils like almond or sesame, because large doses can be toxic and even lethal (read the labels!!!). To skip the worry, just buy scented massage oils in your local bath shops. Choose scents that won't overwhelm, and avoid oils and creams that contain alcohol, because they'll sting—and not in a sexy way. Some of the best rubdown elixirs are those with aloe vera, shea butter, vitamin E, and warming massage oils. The warming sensation will soothe the skin and help both you and your partner relax after all that hard work. With any luck, your massage will be so soothing and sensual that you might be in for the happy ending!

Toys Your Parents Never Gave You

For the ever curious, here is a list of toys that will get you itching for a good spanking!

Feather Tickler: A sultry and seductive way to begin with naughty play, a feather tickler is a sexy, more colorful (and cleaner) version of the French maid variety feather duster. Use it to taunt and tease your partner until he or she is writhing for you!

Riding Crop: Like the ones brandished at the Kentucky Derby, a riding crop is a standard tool for BDSM play. A long rod with a gripping handle, the tip has a small leather fold that will really get your attention on contact.

Plastic or Wooden Cane: Best used for corporal punishment for your lover, a cane is usually lightweight and flexible—it's a tool you can hear coming.

Paddles: There are dozens of different kinds of paddles, which are long, flat pieces of wood (sometimes bound in vinyl or leather) or plastic with short handles. Fur lined paddles give a softer blow; studded paddles pack prickly heat; paddles with holes will bring your swing down with a serious whip; and impression paddles leave marks ranging from cutesy hearts to words like "LOVE" or "SLUT."

Cat o' Nine Tails: A type of flogger, cat o' nine tails have a gripping rod with long leather tails for that feline lashing.

Lash Whip: In the flogging category as well, a lashing whip has a leather handle, often with braided tails that are knotted at the end, with smaller tails stemming from the knots. This whip is for serious BDSM play.

Spanking Gloves: To keep the contact coming, leather spanking gloves will protect your hands from the zing of barehanded blows and boost the impact for your partner. Some gloves are lined with stippling to further exaggerate the sting.

Leather Spanking Skirt: For the spanking seductress, these soft leather skirts are tailored to look like sexy, knee-length pencil skirts from the front, but leave the wearer bare-bottomed in the back for optimal access. Leather straps keep the skirt in place and create a hot bondage look.

Chapter Three

Tie Me Up!

"Thou art to me a
delicious
torment."
—Ralph Waldo Emerson

"Cupid kills with arrows, some with traps."

—Shakespeare
Much Ado about Nothing

INTRODUCTION:
Why Tie?

Playing with ropes with your partner takes a lot of trust, but that can make it even sexier! Part of the fun of bondage is the sense of adventure with a touch of role play. Trussed up and helpless you get to play the damsel in distress, or tie the ropes yourself to play the villain!

The most important element of bondage is the perception of control. Your knots do not have to be flawless: You're not rigging a sailboat, and your partner is not going to drift away on the tide. But you should bind your partner so that it feels real; like good theater, to get the best effect everyone has to play along, but it would be hard to get into the story if the actors had cardboard swords, and you'll feel silly thrashing sexily against uselessly loose bindings. So pick your props with an eye for style, and stick to the scene!

Let's get serious for a second. Sex is awesome, but sex-related accidents are less so. So don't be dumb: Think ahead, and never leave a person tied up alone. Always have a way to free your partner quickly, in case of fire, flood, or zombie apocalypse. Only play tie-up games with partners you trust to untie you, and always respect your partner's boundaries.

Look, No Hands!

THE MOVE

Tying your partner up isn't just supposed to keep him or her still; by binding your partner's wrists, you take away the freedom to use hands for anything at all! Restraining your partner's hands sends a powerful message that you are in control and in charge of what's happening. This message is as visual and symbolic as it is "real," so even with this simple move you have a thousand ways to make it yours.

MAKING IT HAPPEN

Sitting, standing, bent over the couch or propped against the back of an elevator, you can play this game anywhere; the only rule is that for one of you, it's hands-off! Think of this as bondage practice, or the smallest unit of bondage. Simply, one partner loses the use of their hands. You can do this in many ways: While riding on top, hold your partner's hands down with your own, or order your partner to keep the hands above the head on threat of punishment. Of course, for the true bondage feel you need some kind of physical binding—a tie, perhaps?

You can tie wrists together with hands positioned palm to palm, or have the wrists crossed. With palms together, the bound partner can move around and readjust if the bindings become uncomfortable, but some prefer the more elegant look of the crossed wrists. Depending on what activities you have in mind, you can decide to bind hands in front or behind the back. Having your hands bound behind your back can be more challenging than having them tied in front: It affects your balance and makes you more susceptible to falling, all of which also makes you feel more vulnerable (and makes you stick your chest out a bit, which your partner may enjoy as an extra perk!). If you're going to be moving around, it may be easier to keep hands tied in front; that way you are free to help with blow job positioning and flicking hair out of your eyes, but not so free that you have any control. That feeling of helplessness is the flip side of the powerful feeling you get when you tie your partner up, but like we found out with spanking, the partner on top isn't the only one enjoying the game!

Tied Up and Teased

THE MOVE

It's all well and good to say you're going to tie your partner up, but then what? You want to change things up, not just have the same sex you always have with a few extra accessories. You want to make the most of your situation, and the best way to do that is with some well-placed caresses. The goal is twofold: You want to drive your partner crazy with soft strokes that almost—but not quite!—send them off, and you want to flaunt your powerful position by taking your time and putting your hands all over your playmate.

MAKING IT HAPPEN

For this you only need a partner, and something to tie him up with. There are plenty of things you can find around the house for this purpose: scarves, belts, and ties work well, especially to start, as do things like stretchy fabric bandages, fuzzy handcuffs, and so on! Start small until you know what you and your partner are comfortable with. If you decide to use something that fastens or ties securely, like plastic zip ties, rope or cord, make sure you have scissors nearby in case you have to remove the bindings quickly. Wrists and ankles are the most likely parts you'll want to secure, but use caution, since both areas are chock full of sensitive nerves, tendons, and arteries. Don't let your bindings cut off circulation, and if you're going to put any pressure or weight on the bindings, you should spread out the weight by tying multiple points along the same limb. If you're planning to get extra-freaky, you can also buy cuffs and bindings made especially for bondage play, and with safety and style in mind. These come in a variety of materials and types of fastenings. Keep the bindings snug but with a bit of give, so that your partner is comfortable and can wiggle around a little. Your partner might also like to have the bindings positioned so that he has a hand-hold—something to grip in the throes of passion.

Once your partner is securely bound, don't rush to the erogenous zones; instead, touch and kiss your partner slowly along the sternum, all the way down to the abs. This area is very sensitive by its own right, and it has prime real estate right by your partner's naughty bits. Spend some time here, but don't be tempted to move further south: You want to delay gratification for you and your partner, so don't head straight for home plate (or third base... listen, forget sports, just don't let anybody come yet). You can tease with gentle strokes or "accidental" grazes against your partner's sexy parts, but don't linger in any one spot too long. Move slowly, and emphasize your control over the situation by touching your partner in unpredictable patterns and drawing out the foreplay. Remember, this isn't just an excuse to feel your partner up unhindered (although you can certainly do that too): Touch him the way you know he likes it, and if you're not sure where that is, then this is the time to find out! After a bit more teasing, you can take pity on your partner and start dealing out that gratification you've been delaying! Like before, don't spend too long in any one place, but switch up your moves as soon as your partner seems to get used to what you're doing. Once your partner is writhing and ready, you can choose how to finish him off, with a tantalizing blow job, a fast and furious cowgirl romp, or however you'd like—it's up to you!

Bound and Rubbed Down

THE MOVE

Massages are a classic sexy-time move found in even the most vanilla of bedrooms. Rub downs are hot:

The feel of skin on skin, soft moans of pleasure, the physicality of the whole process—all of it is a steamy way to ramp up your tryst. When you add a little bondage to the mix, the combination can be explosive! Just like with the "tie up and tease" move, this trick is all about control. You are in control of your partner's body, and lucky for him or her, you're planning to be nice—for now! You can get a thrill manhandling your helpless partner, and being a bit pushy with your kneading, but the real fun is seeing how many ways you can make your partner beg for more!

MAKING IT HAPPEN

By now you should be a pro at tying your partner up. For this move, it's especially important to keep the bindings loose and comfortable; you want him to pay attention to what you're doing, not be distracted by the rope cutting into his wrist. You can tie your partner lying face-up to start, or find a comfortable way to bind him so you have full access to his back end.

You can set the scene with solid old-school tricks, like lowering the lights, putting on some soft music, and lighting some candles to add needed ambience. Massage oil adds a nice touch as well, or you can use a nice-smelling lotion. And remember that massage oil works on more places than just the back!

To begin, warm up your hands, with or without massage oil, and then gently place your hands on your partner. Pause there for a moment, and then start your massage. Start by kissing your partner, and work your hands behind his head. As you're kissing, gently press your fingers along your partner's spine, starting at the base of his skull. This spot is filled with sensitive nerve endings and pressure points; combined with your kissing, this gentle touch will get you both in the right mindset. Don't spend too much time there, because although it feels heavenly, too much rubbing there can give your partner a headache or leave him sore. As you move further south, concentrate on the bigger muscles like in the arms and shoulders. Make sure to alternate between strong rubbing on the bigger areas and gentle touching on other sensitive places like wrists, hands, and feet. You can get a bit rough (since you're in charge) but be careful not to hurt your partner; a pushy rub-down is hot, a sore muscle or a pinched nerve is not. Pay attention to the noises your partner is making. You know the sounds your partner makes when he's feeling good, so listen for the tell-tale sighs or moans that say you've hit the right spot. You can keep your massage going for as long as you want, then you can decide to end your game by finishing your partner off with your hands, your mouth, or by riding him home.

USING RESTRAINT: TIED DOWN

THE MOVE

There are plenty of ways to tie up your partner, but you can't beat the tried-and-true spread eagle position. It's a comfortable position that doesn't require any strange body contortions, but leaves the bound partner accessible and at your mercy. Lots of the fun of this move comes from the look of the position itself. The perfect picture of the effect of this move can be intense because your hands and feet are bound, but that only makes the end result even more explosive!

MAKING IT HAPPEN

This move is easy for anyone with a big bed with head and footboards, but if your sex cave is still under construction, you can make a few changes to get any bedroom a-rocking. You can buy cheap drawer handles, or even just a few eye hooks, and secure them to your bed frame or the wall behind your bed, in suitable "spread eagle" placements. You may not want to do this if you're afraid of being found out, but the small hooks shouldn't be too noticeable depending on where you install them. For a much more subtle option, you can invest in a set of specially-made bondage sheets with anchors for straps built right in, or you can get a similar effect by running some rope or bungee cord underneath your mattress. Get creative and you should be able to find a good solution for your situation.

Whether by hook or by headboard, your next step is to tie 'em down. Each hand is tied separately to the bed or hook, and the ankles are secured with the legs spread apart. If you're being tied up, make sure you're comfortable, because you'll be here a while! With this move the bound partner has even less physical control over the situation, which can be seriously heady! Remember, even though you are tied down, you can help control the action with verbal cues. This is especially fun and helpful as you're starting out, because you have to think about and put into words what you want and where you want it. Once you get more comfortable you can change the rules, and let your partner find his own way to drive you crazy.

PLAYING ALONG: TIED SITTING

THE MOVE

Sex tied to the bed is exciting, but it's still . . . sex in a bed. There are plenty of other pieces of furniture around your house that you can use to strap in! Chairs are great and give you a different experience from being tied to the bed—the restrained partner is sitting up and can look around while still being securely tied up.

MAKING IT HAPPEN

There are a few ways to tie someone to a chair, and they mostly depend on what chair you have in mind. Kitchen chairs usually have plenty of slats and dowels to tie things to, and are made of solid wood or other materials that are easy to clean after the fun. If your chair has arms, they make good places to secure the bound partner's wrists, but this configuration can limit access and movement more than you'd like. With an armless chair, you can have your wrists tied behind your back or secured to the sides of the chair. Securing the feet is easy: Ankles can be tied to the chair legs or each other, with the knees pushed

The only way to
get rid of a
temptation
is to
yield to it."

—Oscar Wilde
The Picture of
Dorian Gray

together or pulled wide, depending on what you have planned! When playing around with bondage and smaller furniture like chairs, make sure that the chair is on a solid surface and watch that it doesn't fall over during your sexcapade.

Since the sitting position gives your partner a good view, use this to your advantage and put on a show. You have an audience, so enjoy it. You can put on a sexy lap dance or striptease, or don a costume or sexy accessories and enjoy the fact that your partner can only look, not touch! Unlike earlier moves where you wanted your touches to be surprising and unexpected, here you want to telegraph your touches, to let your partner know "I'm going to touch you here . . . because I said so!"

The downside of the chair position is that it limits access to most of the sexy bits, especially if the bound partner is of the vagina-having variety. You can get around this by relegating the chair to foreplay, and activating your ejector button (or just untying the knots) before you both finish, or you can go the distance by getting creative and a little flexible. If your partner is a guy, your job's a bit easier. You can give him a toe-curling blow job, and he's got a front-row seat. If your chair is sturdy, you can climb on board and enjoy some hot face-to-face chair sex.

On Your Knees

THE MOVE

Bondage is about power and control, so what better way to show that than with some bondage keeping you on your knees? Kneeling is a powerful symbol of submission, so this move will be extra-thrilling for the bound partner, who gets to play at being helpless and dominated, and for the dominating partner, who enjoys this display of subservience from a higher, more powerful position.

MAKING IT HAPPEN

There are many ways to bind your partner kneeling. You don't have to do a full-body binding—you can use the techniques discussed earlier to bind your partner's wrists, commanding them to kneel, or guiding/physically positioning them with your hands. This kind of external power play can be extra sexy paired with the submissive position. If you want the full bondage solution, you can try a variation on the Hog Tie position, which I'll talk more about later. For this move, have the bound partner kneel in a comfortable position, with hands at his or her sides.

Then tie each wrist to the corresponding ankle (left to left, etc.), leaving enough rope so that the bound partner can still kneel comfortably, but not so loose that they can use the hands. This position can make the bound partner lose balance, and with the hands bound he or she won't be able to stop a fall, so keep a supportive hand on your partner, and never leave him or her alone.

The kneeling position is nice to look at, and it puts the bound partner at just about the perfect height to perform some oral sex. If you have trouble making that work comfortably with the bound partner kneeling and the other standing, try using different chairs or sitting on the edge of the bed. However you make it work, this move hits you with a double-whammy of hot visuals and good positioning.

FANCY ROPE WORK

THE MOVE

If ropes have gotten your motor running, you're in luck! There's an almost endless number of ways to tie someone up, as long as you have enough rope and a willing partner. Different bondage configurations work for different kinds of games and positions. In all cases, the fun is in the power play, but also partly in the theater of the game. Advanced bondage steps up the intensity on both fronts: With these tricks the partner on top has more control, and the partner set to be tied has even less, and less chance of movement, as well. Advanced rope work often also looks cooler, and more intense, which multiplies the effect. These tricks come with the same warnings as before: Be smart, use common sense, and don't ever leave your partner tied up alone. Because these tricks involve more rope covering more of your body, they can be a tad more dangerous than beginner moves. But when you're playing safely, these ramped-up moves can make your sex sesh incredibly kinky and fun!

MAKING IT HAPPEN

Hog Tie:

You've probably heard the term "hogtied" before, since it's a pretty common term that people use to simply mean "tied up completely." In this case, hogtying is a specific rope arrangement where the person's wrists and ankles are fastened, and drawn together with another binding, either in front or behind the back. This position makes it impossible for the bound partner to move. First, bind your partner's wrists together, then the ankles. Then grab another rope and run it through (or otherwise connect it to) the bindings around the wrists and ankles. Adjust the connector rope to pull the wrists and ankles closer together, only as much as is comfortable. Now review your work—you have a neatly-tied gift laid out in front of you! You may not actually be able to have sex with your partner in this position, but it works great for foreplay, or for dom/sub role-play.

Frogtie:

The frogtie is a more utilitarian version of the hog tie that gives you access to the bound partner's sexy bits, allowing you to use this position during oral sex, while playing with toys, and a whole bunch of other fun activities. There are variations to this move. The more advanced technique involves tying one's ankles to the calves, right at the hip, so that the knees are kept bent (like a frog's, apparently) and the bound are unable to move. The simpler way to accomplish this move is to fasten each wrist to the corresponding ankle. This gives the bound partner more wiggle room than the trickier version, but it's also more comfortable and easier to accomplish. This technique is great because it works for a bunch of different positions. The bound partner can lie down, with her arms by her side, which pulls her ankles back and apart, or she can sit up or be propped up against a headboard.

A more grueling version of this is the Leapfrog position. Essentially this is the frogtie with the bound partner lying face down. It can become painful quickly, so don't plan to spend too much time in this position, since it puts so much strain on the neck and shoulders. To accomplish this position, have the bound partner kneel on the bed, (if you're doing this somewhere other than the bedroom, make sure the surface you're on is soft and comfortable, or this will hurt!). Pull each arm down and between the legs, and fasten it to the corresponding ankle (right to right, etc.). When that's done, the bound partner will be lying with her head and shoulders pressed against the bed, with her ass in the air. This is a hot position for spanking or rear-entry, and it just plain looks sexy!

The Ball Tie:

This position is so simple and easy to do, and works with so many different sex positions, that it's a wonder that it hasn't gained more notoriety. Lay back on the bed, then pull your knees up to your chest, like you're curling up into a ball. Wrap your arms around your legs, and have your partner secure your wrists together. Voila! With one small binding you are now an incapacitated ball of sex, you sexy thing, you! This position leaves your ass and sexy bits exposed, making this trick perfect for pre-spanking bondage.

MORE BINDING OPTIONS

N ow that I've shown you the ropes, feel free to get creative with some other exciting bondage equipment. That old tie you've been using is getting a bit ratty....

Leather

Leather bindings are both comfortable and sturdy, with a nice sheen and a look that means business. Accessories can make a big difference in bondage play, since it helps you get into the spirit of the game, so bringing leather into your bed can be extra kinky!

Basic leather gear includes leather cuffs, collars, and other more mainstream sexy garments like bustiers and corsets. These can be useful in bondage play, since they often have straps that make them easy to fasten to other things. The real perk of leather accessories is the look: Leather is just sexy. And since it's the look you want, if you or your partner is vegan you can find all sorts of classy faux-leather online.

Metal

Metal bonds are useful because they are strong, sturdy, and tend to be latched or fastened in a way that makes them easy to put on and remove quickly. Metal bindings, like handcuffs, can be less comfortable than softer bindings, and they may leave marks if the bound partner pulls against them, so keep that in mind when you plan your scenes.

Metal bindings are fairly basic. You have the typical wrist cuffs and ankle cuffs, along with the more exotic thumb cuffs. You can also find "fuzzy" cuffs, which are lined with some other material to make them more comfortable. For more advanced play, you can find bars and spreaders to hold apart the bound partner's ankles, or to bind their arms, like stocks. Metal, like leather, is used for its looks: Metal bindings are hard, cold, and unyielding, making this material well suited for a rougher tumble.

Rope

There are a ton of different kinds of rope you can use for bondage play, and there are even more kinds of rope that are *not* for bondage. You can find rope at most home improvement stores (if you have to ask, just say you're building a tire swing or something—you may want to leave this book at home). Find a rope that's soft on your skin, and that can hold a knot. Materials like cotton, nylon, or hemp are a good bet. If you're looking for something rougher, look for sisal rope or some other natural fiber. While you're at the store, you may want to look for eye hooks or anchors you can attach to your bed to make for some fun rope configurations.

Other Stuff

If you really want to play with bondage, you can get almost anything you need from a sex store online. Yeah, you can play with stuff you have, but the best accessories are the ones that were made for the job. Two great tools you can get are velcro straps and bondage tape.

Velcro straps are quick to secure, like leather or metal cuffs, but they're a whole lot more comfortable. With straps, you can try out positions that were too difficult to tie on your own. You can get wrist and ankle straps, which work like cuffs, or straps designed for a specific position, like hog tie straps.

Bondage tape is great, and it's the only kind of tape you should ever use for bondage, because it's specially made to be put on skin. Other types of tape, especially something strong like duct tape, can be difficult to remove safely; bondage tape, though, can be used as a binding, as a blindfold, or almost anything you want.

Chapter 4

Turn Me On!

"That I may see her
   and feel her nearness,
which produces an effect
on me like poetry,
   like music."

—Ritter von Leopold Sacher-Masoch
Venus in Furs

"When I see a
pretty pair of calves
in silk stockings it
makes me long to
look higher..."

—Anonymous
"Miss Coote's Confession"
(From The Pearl)

S ight, sound, smell, taste, and touch—we use our senses every day to explore the world around us. So when you take away senses, or change them, it affects how we experience everything, including sex! This chapter is all about manipulating your senses to have amazing, mind-blowing sex. This technique is sometimes called sensation play, because the focus is on what you're feeling, and how you're feeling it. This chapter will tell you all about some fun, kinky classics, like the basics of blindfolding, how to use ice and hot wax, and some more advanced techniques like using Ben Wa balls and sex with headphones!

BASICS OF BLINDFOLDING

THE MOVE

Being blindfolded is one of the simplest sexy tricks you can add to your romp. While blindfolded, you're not distracted by your overfull laundry pile or the time on the alarm clock. You're free to focus on the pleasure of the moment. Blindfolding is also a form of sensory deprivation, where you are deprived of one sense in order to strengthen the others. Think about when you walk through a dark room: You have no choice but to concentrate on your surroundings and reach out to feel for objects in your path. Even if you've walked through that room ten times that day, it is a different experience in the dark. It is the same way with sex blindfolded. Add to that the element of surprise—you never know where or when you'll be touched—and this basic is a big win.

MAKING IT HAPPEN

Blindfolds are easy to find. You can use a soft scarf, a bit of fabric, a t-shirt, or a sleep mask—as long as it's comfortable and stays secured for most of the festivities. Once you find your chosen accessory, secure it in front of your partner's eyes. It should be snug, comfortable, and not block his or her breathing.

Your blindfolded partner should then lie back as you begin. With his sight now gone, your partner will be even more sensitive to your touches, so use this dynamic to your advantage! Tease him with light, unexpected touches all across his body, paying attention to erogenous zones around his ears and neck, his nipples, and down to his genitals. He won't be able to see where you plan on touching him next or how, so be unpredictable and use light, soft touches. As you tease your partner, pay attention to how he responds and moves, and follow his lead. Use your mouth to add more sensations, trailing kisses down his stomach or sucking gently on his earlobe before blowing a shiver-inducing breath of air across his neck. As you and your partner climb closer to orgasm, you can choose to take the mask off, or ride your masked partner into the sunset . . .

AURAL SEX

THE MOVE

Music and sex go together like wine and cheese (or maybe wine and sex?), but this move ramps it up to the next level. With this move, you use a pair of headphones and a carefully selected playlist to block all outside noise. Like with the blindfold, it works through sensory deprivation and the power of a good rhythm. Paired with a blindfold, this move can be a thousand shades of orgasmic—with a capital O.

MAKING IT HAPPEN

Your first step is to choose a song, and set it up to play from a set of headphones. Choose the song your partner will listen to, and make sure it fits the tone you want to set. This move works with slow, sensual tunes and fast hip-grinding beats; just make sure your fucking fits the tempo! Once you choose a song and prepare the electronics, you're ready to go. Blindfold your partner as instructed above, and then have him put on the headphones and start the music, setting the song on repeat or looping a play-list. Your partner is now even more sensory-deprived and focused on your touch, and farther away from distractions. Start teasingly, like you did with the blindfold; with all of his attention on you, a little touch goes a long way. Use your fingers to lightly scratch down his chest, pressing your nails into him, but without leaving a mark. Use your mouth to kiss or suck other sensitive parts of his body, like on the inside of his hip, and surprise him with a quick swirl of your tongue around the head of his penis. Once you are ready, straddle him and slide him inside of you. Move your body rhythmically along with the music, keeping up with your light touches and soft strokes, until the song—and you and your partner— reach a crescendo.

Be sure to switch places for an encore!

PLAYTIME PLAYLIST

Here are some songs to get you started on your aural adventure! If none of these curl your toes, try some other types of stimulating sounds, like a ticking metronome, some lyricless classical music, or a tune with a pounding bass.

Madonna "Justify My Love"

Bruce Springsteen "I'm on Fire"

TLC "Red Light Special"

Boys II Men "I'll Make Love to You"

Katy Perry "Dressin' Up"

Foo Fighters "Everlong"

Janet Jackson "The Velvet Rope"

Nine Inch Nails "Closer"

Aaliyah "Rock the Boat"

The Cars "Who's Gonna Drive You Home"

Garbage "#1 Crush"

The Black Keys "The Only One"

Next "Too Close"

Deftones "Passenger"

Usher "Love in this Club"

Marvin Gaye "Let's Get it On"

Barry White "Can't get Enough of Your Love"

Rub Up Against Me

THE MOVE

Another way to play with sensations is to bring different textures into play! Fabrics or materials can create different sensations as they are rubbed, dragged, or flicked onto your body, and you can use a variety of materials to get just the right reaction from your

"My tongue is useless;
   A subtle fire
    Runs through my body;
My eyes are sightless,
And my ears ringing"

—Sappho

partner. This works especially well when your or your partner's senses are heightened from sensory deprivation.

MAKING IT HAPPEN

Gather a variety of different materials; some old favorites include soft materials like silk and fur, as well as feathers, in or out of a duster. These and other soft materials like fleece or fine cotton feel soft and sensual, so use them to gently stroke your partner's sensitive erogenous zones. Be a tease: Use a feather or silk to trace a path down your partner's torso, drawing circles around his abdomen.

You can also use rougher materials for a different kind of sensation. Use leather or wool gloves to stroke your partner's chest or cheek, or just to grip his arm. Try other materials you have around the house, like denim, terrycloth, and jersey, to see what works for you.

Brushes are a great tool for this, too, and you probably have a bunch of different kinds around the house already. Paint brushes, hair brushes, even tooth brushes can be used to great effect on the most sensitive areas of your partner.

ICY HOT

THE MOVE

Ice is a great seduction tool, especially when things get hot. The cold gives you a shock, leaves a wide trail of cold water down your back, and then where it settles it burns until you can dig it out. This same mix of feelings—the shock, the chill of an icy water trail, and the burn of a settled ice cube—is why using ice during sex is so hot. Ice can stimulate sensitive spots all over your body or you can use the ice to cool your mouth for another cool treat! Using ice during sex is even steamier when you play the heat of your bodies against the chill of the ice.

MAKING IT HAPPEN

Start with an ice cube. It may help to run it under water after you take it out of the freezer, so it doesn't stick to your skin. Have your partner lie down and start by putting the ice cube in your mouth. Trail your chilled lips across his chest, down his stomach to his penis. Slip him inside your mouth and let him feel the temperature change. Once your mouth has warmed, slide him out slowly and blow on him gently to give him another sexy cold shiver. Now that he's warmed up, cool him off by trailing the ice slowly across his body. Focus on sensitive erogenous areas like his wrists, behind his ear, even his feet. Remember to keep the ice moving to keep the sensation light and exciting—focusing on one spot too long can leave your lover more chilly than turned on! As you move the ice around his body, follow it with your mouth, using kisses and flicks of the tongue to temper the cold ice with your warm mouth.

Ice play doesn't need to be limited to just using cubes—try freezing water into a large straw to make a tantalizing ice wand. To hit a real icy peak, freeze water inside a condom supported by a paper towel roll or other household item, and create your own ice dildo that will leave you and your partner shivering for more!

Waxing Poetic: Using Hot Wax

THE MOVE

Dripping hot wax—the image alone is hot and kinky. As with ice play, the fun of playing with wax comes

"In this garden all the hot noon
I await thy fluttering footfall
Through the twilight."

—Sappho

from the new, exciting sensations and temperature changes. It's important to be careful when you're playing with fire, but using hot wax is safe . . . and smoking hot.

MAKING IT HAPPEN

Many sex shops sell candles just for this purpose; you can even get candles that melt at a lower temperature. Try using paraffin wax, but steer clear from scented, or even colored candles, which have chemicals that may cause irritation. You can also start out using a birthday candle—they have less wax, so they are easier to manage, especially for a beginner. It's best to start slow with wax, gradually getting used to the feeling of hot wax dripping or being spread on your body. You can begin by burning the candle until you get a small pool of wax. Dip your finger in the pool, coating it with wax, then dip it again into the melted candle so that more hot wax is stuck to the tip. Slowly move your finger to your partner's body, tracing lines and swirls on her skin. This technique is gentle, so it can be used on sensitive areas like nipples once your partner is comfortable with the temperature and sensation.

When you both feel comfortable, you can try dripping wax directly onto your partner.

Start by pouring or dripping the wax into your partner's hand. If she enjoys that, you can move on to drip wax onto her thighs and legs, back, or ass cheeks. You can vary the feeling of the wax by dripping it from different distances, or by blowing on the wax gently before it drips. Dripping from higher up will cool down the wax before it hits the skin, which can help to avoid burns. You can also peel the wax off quickly after dripping it, and use your mouth to cool the hot skin. There are many options for personalizing this move, so play around with your partner! Just remember to make it *hot* . . . but not too hot!

BEN WA BALLS

THE MOVE

This accessory has been around for ages, and goes by many different names, including Venus Balls, Geisha Balls, or to cut to the chase, Orgasm Balls. You can find this toy where fine sex toys are sold, or on the internet! Ben Wa balls are a set of two small, weighted balls, often connected by a string or thread, that you insert into the vagina. These balls can be used

"The man should do whatever the girl takes most delight in, and should get for her whatever she may want. So he should bring her such playthings as may be hardly known to other girls. He may show her a ball dyed with various colors, and other curiosities like that."

—Vātsyāyana.
Kama Sutra

for exercise and pleasure. To keep them from falling out, you, or the lady in question, have to flex the PC muscles, strengthening them in much the same way as Kegel exercises. But that's not why you should run out and buy them! The shape of the balls and the weights inside them make the Ben Wa balls move and roll in a way that stimulates a woman in a new, exciting way. The feeling is intensified when you move around, and the...portable...nature of this toy makes for plenty of sexy opportunities.

MAKING IT HAPPEN

First, lubricate the balls either with some personal lubricant or with your mouth. Carefully and gently slide them into the vagina. Once they are inserted, test out how they feel by having her stand up and walk a bit. Once the Ben Wa balls feel comfortable, you or your partner can try "wearing" them around the house, doing chores or going about everyday business—taking sexy games out of the bedroom can be unbelievably exciting.

There are plenty of moves and activities you and your partner can use to get the most out of your Ben Wa balls. Almost any movement that will make the balls move and roll will create new, interesting, and toe-curling sensations. Try sex positions or other movements involving rocking, like spanking, or use a vibrator. Ben Wa balls create a unique effect, so test them out and see what works for you.

Show Me Your Teeth

THE MOVE

Biting is a good beginner technique as it needs hardly any props, and it is an easy way to deal out some pain—but not too much! Biting taps into the primal side of sex, and has always been a sign of passion— the practice, and the marks it leaves.

MAKING IT HAPPEN

Start your sensual biting with some sensual kissing. Once things have gotten hot and heavy, begin to gently nibble on your partner's lips, then slowly sweep down to graze your teeth over your partner's lips and jaw. Work your way downward, nipping your partner top to bottom—you want to devour your partner! Concentrate on the erogenous zones, nipping (gently!) at his neck and ears, down to his hips and genitals. Make sure not to spend too long in one spot—nibbling and teeth-grazing is hot, gnawing is not.

FIELD TRIP: SEX IN ALMOST-PUBLIC PLACES

THE MOVE

Part of the fun in playing with sensations is that you get to experience sex in a whole new way. Stepping outside your comfort zone can be thrilling and make your sex even better. So where do you go once you've had wild, blindfolded sex on every surface in your house? Outside!

MAKING IT HAPPEN

The most difficult part of this move is finding a good spot outdoors. Sex in a phone booth on a busy street sounds exciting, but misdemeanor charges are not. Instead, try out almost-public spaces that will still make you feel naughty and get that blood pumping for when it counts. If you're lucky, you have a big fenced in yard with no nosy neighbors. If not, you'll have to get creative. Once you've found your grassy knoll, spread out a blanket and get busy. While you do, pay attention to the smell of the grass, the sound of the birds, and the feel of wind on your skin. The new environment and the chance of getting caught in the act will all heighten your sexual high.

Chapter Five:

Submission

"Poor Louisa, however,
bore up at length
better than could have
been expected: and though
she suffered, and
greatly too, yet,
ever true to the good
old cause, she suffered
with pleasure and
enjoyed her pain."

—John Cleland
Memoirs Of Fanny Hill

"I snatchted her gown:
being thin, the harm
   was small,
   Yet strived she
to be covered there withal.
And striving thus as
   one would be cast,
Betrayde herself,
   and yielded at the last."

—Ovid
Elegy 5

INTRO:
About Submitting

⌒〜

To some, taking on the submissive role sounds like the result of a lost bet. The submissive, or "bottom," is expected to be obedient in a BDSM relationship, assuming whatever role, or accepting whatever punishment his or her partner demands. Some relationships even continue this beyond the bedroom, where submissives are "slaves," or more clearly, they are consensually under the ownership of their partners, who decide various parameters of the submissives' behavior. While this kind of submission is extreme, you can explore the dynamics of submission by being held down or tied up.

When compared with the other puzzle piece, the dominant, the mere sound of being the "submissive" automatically makes it sound like it sucks. Fear not! Being the submissive is actually incredibly sexy—both because your body is chemically inclined to like it, and because in a society where upward mobility is the name of the game, lying back and taking it can feel so good. This chapter will explore why we find pleasure in a little bit of pain, and the secret no one wants you to know: Being submissive actually puts you in control. If you find that you have trouble behaving, a few obedience tips will help keep you in line the next time you find yourself tied, tickled, or tamed. Do yourself a favor and submit!

Why Being Submissive is Hot:
The Pleasure of Pain

SPANKER'S HIGH

As a submissive, your dominant may ask you to do a full range of things during a particularly spicy tumble in bed, whether it's introducing your bare buns to an eager studded paddle, testing out those sailing knots, or taunting you with candle wax. If you've never tried any of these things out, the fear of a little bit of pain can be intimidating. Luckily, your body has natural defenses for taking these doses of discomfort and converting them into a euphoric high.

When you experience pain, whether it's stubbing your toe, cutting your finger, or getting spanked by your lover for being naughty, your brain releases endorphins, which are chemicals that connect with opiate receptors in your brain to minimize how you experience pain. They create feelings of euphoria and lower stress levels, functioning in much the same way as drugs like morphine and codeine (without the pesky drug addiction). This is where the term "runner's high," comes from, in that when people exercise, their brains release endorphins to distract from the exhaustion from physical activity—consider it nature's way of rewarding you for going to the gym. Certain foods are known to release endorphins as well. Unsurprisingly, chocolate is one of them—but chili peppers are, too! This is why some people love spicy foods; they know they're in for serious heat, but as they bite into that pepper and get the first bursts of spice and pain, their bodies are simultaneously producing endorphins to soothe and excite, which makes people come back for more.

Being on the receiving end of a little punishment is just like munching on chili peppers. It's spicy and a little bit nerve-wracking beforehand, but your body is prepared for it. Getting spanked during a sexy session with your dominant gives your body more reasons to produce the good kind of chemicals, which can lead to an even more powerful climax.

WHAT THE DOCTOR ORDERED

The act of submission is exceptionally cathartic, relieving tension and stress, and even feelings of guilt. The average person's buildup of stress—whether from work, family, finances, or otherwise—can be overwhelming at best. Where some people choose stress reducers like cardio, yoga, or compulsively refreshing their online bank statements to make sure their bills have cleared, others go with the, "Fuck me and make it hurt," approach.

Relieving built up tension is a huge part of the success of taking on the submissive role. People talk about how phenomenal makeup sex is in this way. Besides the whole, "I love you and nothing can keep us apart," aspect, this is because more often than not, you're still kind of pissed off at the person and are able to transfer your frustration into a particularly steamy and aggressive sexual romp. Makeup sex is good for the relationship, but it's also good for blowing off steam. This is how some of your submissive scenes can play out, and it's an amazing way to test your limits. There's something liberating about knowing how hard you can have your hair pulled, your lip bit, or your ass smacked during sex with your partner. Having your partner hold you down while you struggle for your reward makes that reward all the more thrilling once it's given to you.

BDSM is aggressive physical activity at its peak, which gives your body something to focus on other than whatever stress is currently weighing you down. And it's okay that this kind of intense physical activity leaves a mark. Just like getting hickeys as a teenager, physical reminders of these sessions—like a bright red handprint on your backside, or some bruising where you were tied up—are naughty little trophies for the hours or days following your sexcapades.

HOW BEING ON THE BOTTOM GIVES YOU THE UPPER HAND

In a society where compliance is a dirty word, especially for women in the work force, being sexually submissive sounds like a kick in the shins to self-actualization and the women's movement. Not so! The reality is that in the twenty-first century, women are more and more becoming the breadwinners in their families, and represent 60% of those pursuing higher education. For both men and women, meeting goals and deadlines, buying a house, and providing for 2.5 kids and a golden retriever is all the dominance they need. Most among the hardworking task force have no greater fantasy than to just relax on a beach and do nothing—this fantasy isn't so far off from submission. Being sexually submissive allows you—whether male or female—to put aside difficult choices and the position of authority you have to assert on a daily basis. It's about being pleasured in an unconventional way by someone you trust.

Submission is sexually invigorating and therapeutic in the same way that role-playing fulfills fantasies you would otherwise not experience. In simple terms: Powerful men and women still want to be dominated. Gender roles used to insist that men be rugged, handy, and bring home the bacon, while women be sweet, feminine, and take care of the family. Now, gender roles expect that both genders do all of these things, mixing and matching, depending on the situation. Women should be powerful, pull themselves up by their bootstraps, work 40+ hours a week, and be caring wives and mothers. Men should also be powerful, pull themselves up by their bootstraps, work 40+ hours a week, and be conscientious husbands and fathers. This is an enormous amount of responsibility when considering that modern media continues to hurl conflicting expectations via cosmetic ads, airbrushed magazine covers, and reality television, ultimately confusing the shit out of you about how you're supposed to act. For these reasons, it's totally okay to want to be the business exec publicly, and slutty Susie Homemaker inside closed doors (or vice versa!). It is in no way an emasculating swat to your manhood or a degrading swipe to your female empowerment to want to be dominated.

In a submissive-dominant relationship, one of the sexiest things for the dominant is knowing that his or her submissive is conceding to certain nasty little desires in order to please. This doesn't mean that wanting to please is a one-way street, and a huge misconception about submission is that the sub has no power. True: As the bottom, you're going to be

"You know nothing gives
me greater happiness
than to **serve you,**
to be **your slave.**
I would give everything
for the sake
of feeling myself
wholly in your power,
even unto death."

—Leopold Sacher-Masoch
Venus in Furs

told what to do with that ice dildo and how many times to do it. False: You can't say no to the ice dildo, the riding crop, or the nipple clamps, and your wants don't matter. Quite the contrary, the submissive has the most control—perhaps not mid-throes, but definitely when lines are being drawn in the sand and limits are reached. The submissive always has veto power. Most couples make hard and soft limits very clear before going down any roads paved with floggers and chains. The sub is allowed to expressly prohibit any toys, activities, or invasions of personal boundaries. This also goes for knowing when to stop. It might be sexy as hell to count with your partner how many times he or she has smacked you with a lash-whip while you get it on, but when enough is enough, your dominant must stop when you say so. While your partner may fine-tune the details of how you receive your punishments and your rewards, as the submissive, you control the context.

OBEDIENCE TIPS

Being your dominant's naughty little girl or bad little boy requires attention to detail, endurance, and naturally, the eagerness to please. While it may be the dominant partner's job to keep the submissive in line, there are ways that the sub can harness the reins a little to fully explore his or her role as the bottom. Learning what works for you and your partner in your BDSM fantasies will improve the quality of each feisty encounter. Follow this general guide to obedience every time you find yourself stepping a toe out of line—unless, of course, you want to be punished!

SET RULES

First and foremost, you need to set rules with your dominant. Working up a 60-page contract works for some, while others are okay with sticking to Scout's Honor. Within these rules, you can confirm or deny the requests of your dominant, and clearly lay out how, when, and where your lusty liaisons will occur, if you so choose. Setting rules ensures that you and your partner can explore one another's curiosities without feeling uncomfortable.

HAVE A SAFEWORD

Choosing a safeword is to rough, kinky sex as landing gear is to a 747. It's really fucking important. Choose a word that is completely unrelated to the context, and one that your dominant won't mistakenly interpret as dirty talk or role-playing. Largely, words like "no," "stop," or "that hurts" can be confusing; if you're handcuffed to the bed as a high-security prisoner who needs corporal punishment, these words will only give you more of what you're getting. If you're a visual learner, elect "red" for "Stop, I've had enough," "yellow" for "Slow down or ease up," and "green" for "Hit me, baby!" If you're feeling creative, choose a family of nouns that will give the automatic signal for your partner to change what he or she is doing, whether it's "grizzly bear," "panda," and "koala" for stop, ease up, and go; or "Chris Brown," "Kanye," and "Justin Bieber." If you'd rather keep it simple and use "no," or "stop," just be clear that these words have to be obeyed. Whatever you choose, make sure these words are set in stone and memorized by all.

HIT THE GYM

Sweaty sex is super hot, but sweaty sex where you start wheezing, take time-outs to prevent an impending coronary, and fall flaccid is not. Not only will you feel more confident about being naked in front of your partner, but eating healthy and doing a little bit of cardio a handful of times a week will improve your endurance and longevity when it really counts.

If "running" is one of your curse words, try going for brisk walks after meals, swimming, biking, or virtually any sport or activity that gets your blood flowing for more than twenty minutes each time. You'll thank yourself when your partner introduces the sex swing.

DOMINATE YOUR SUBMISSION

Own it! Being a submissive may sound like an easy gig, but just because you're the bottom doesn't mean you get to act like a dead fish. Enthusiastically taking on your role as a sub is hard work, both physically and emotionally. Knowing this is half the battle, and the other half is doing your best to reach the goals you've set with your partner. If being the sub works for you, then revel in it! Provoke the hit from the "SLUT" paddle, tempt the cane, and invite the handcuffs. Eagerly anticipating each rough rendezvous will pay off tenfold for both you and your dom.

YOUR BEDROOM BOOK CLUB

↶

A s long as there have been humans, there has been sex, and as long as there has been literature, there has been erotic literature. Be well-read in these classic erotic tales and spice up your sex life—whether it's with a partner, or on your own.

Kama Sutra by Vātsyāyana

This is the sex gold standard. Written by the ancient Indian Hindu philosopher Vātsyāyana, this book provides a breadth of practical sex advice and tantalizing positions for him and her, but also offers poetry and a guide to virtuous living, love, and family.

Anaïs Nin

Anaïs Nin was a French Cuban writer who was one of the first women to explore erotic fiction. Much of her work was written in the 1940s, but published posthumously. In collections of short stories such as, "Delta of Venus" (1978) and "Little Birds" (1979), Nin delves into an array of modes of sexuality, including topics controversial for the time like abuse, prostitution, and bisexuality.

Sleeping Beauty Trilogy by Anne Rice

The Claiming of Sleeping Beauty (1983), *Beauty's Punishment* (1984) and *Beauty's Release* (1985) make up Anne Rice's trilogy loosely adapted on the Sleeping Beauty fairy tale, with a BDSM twist.

The Story of O by Pauline Réage

This French BDSM novel, published in 1954, was a controversial story about a beautiful Parisian girl who is thrown deep into the world of submission, bondage, and pain play.

Tropic of Cancer by Henry Miller

This novel by one of America's most famous and revered writers was originally published in France in 1934—but banned in the U.S. When it was finally released in America in 1961, it led to obscenity trials. If that's not enough of a reason to read it, it's also considered a masterpiece of American literature. And it takes place in Paris.

Lady Chatterley's Lover by D. H. Lawrence

Originally published in 1928, this novel's heroine, Constance (Lady Chatterly), marries into high society, but finds herself in a lusty tryst with a working-class man. Considered taboo for its explicit scenes and abundant use of the word "fuck," this novel was banned for years.

Chapter Six

Domination

"A girl who is much
    sought after should marry
the man that she likes,
and whom she thinks
    would be obedient
    to her, and capable
of giving her pleasure."

—Vātsyāyana
Kama Sutra

"Love is the fulfilling of the law."

—Romans 13:10

INTRODUCTION:
Be the Boss

THE MOVE

Let out your inner dom—leather and studs optional! Playing the dom, or "top," is a challenge: You plan the games, do all of the heavy lifting, and keep a constant eye on your partner and the situation to make sure that everyone is safe, happy, and having fun. But of course, all of this work comes with some very real perks! Playing the dominant can be fun for people who already like being bossy, and it can also provide a new experience and outlet for someone who isn't used to barking orders.

Domination and submission is all about the game of power, and when you play the dom, you have all of the power. What you do with that power is up to you: You can show your partner just how much pleasure you can give him, or be selfish and command your sub to serve you. So put on (or take off?) your bossypants and get started!

MAKING IT HAPPEN

Dominance/ submission is sort of like any other sexy role-playing game you bring into your bedroom: You have to get into the spirit of the game for it to work. What that means is up to you and your partner, since there's no "right" way to play. That doesn't mean you have to be all serious and dungeon-master-y, but you do want to feel powerful, and for your partner to feel that you're in control.

With all of the whips and chains and black leather, the dom often seems like the bad guy of the BDSM world, but that's not quite right. Remember that you aren't the villain in this scene, but the figure of authority. You're not being "mean" to your partner, you're just taking charge.

The best way to do that is to plan. The old advice is that sex should be spontaneous, spur of the moment, driven by passion. But to play dominant most effectively, you need to have a plan, if only so you can tell your partner, "Ooh baby, wait until you see what I have planned for you!"

Don't ask what your partner wants—this breaks the power dynamic you've set up, and doesn't really give your partner the submissive experience he or she is looking for. If you're just starting out, or trying something new and you're not sure how your partner will like it, you can ask "do you want me to . . . (do XYZ)," or simply tell your partner "I'm going to do this to you!" and pay attention to his response, both what he says and what his body language tells you.

THE CARE AND KEEPING OF SUBS

THE MOVE

Most of the focus is one-sided. The dominant partner is usually the active one, whereas the submissive is typically acted on. Everything is usually hunky-dory in BDSM land, but how can make sure it stays that way? Since you're playing with power dynamics, things can get complicated fast, and it's your responsibility as the head honcho to create a fun space for you and your partner to safely explore new feelings and push boundaries. You need to build trust with your partner—this is a new-ish kind of trust, because your sub needs to trust that you don't intend to hurt her, *and* that you are skilled enough that you know how to keep her safe. These tips can help reassure both of you on both counts. You may think that these tips will be more helpful for more advanced players, but the basics can help you and your partner avoid bruised wrists and hurt feelings, even if you're not suspending anyone from the ceiling.

Talk about it First:

You probably don't need to draft a contract before you break out the blindfold, but before you try anything adventurous in bed, you're going to want to talk it over. Just as some people can't walk and chew gum at the same time, you might find it difficult to have a frank, honest talk about sex while you're actually doing it. So before you get naked, talk about it. Think about what you want and don't want during sex, go over boundaries, and be specific. If you've never really thought about this stuff before, this exercise can be enlightening.

This chat isn't a one-time discussion, either. Communication is vital to good sex, and so important to keeping BDSM play safe and fun. Check in with your partner, and ask questions when you're not sure if he or she likes what you're doing.

Once you've gone over boundaries and talked about what turns you on, you both have a much better idea of where your partner stands. The talk is just to set up guidelines, not to give one partner the green light to tie the other up and try out all of the things she didn't say "no" to.

Which brings us to . . .

Safe Words

Safe words were an early kink artifact picked up by the mainstream, so most people at least know the general idea behind them. You may think that you don't need a safe word in your loving, trusting, kinky-sex-having relationship, but they can be useful for a few reasons. Having a safe word can crank up the erotic factor, and help you better understand what your partner needs and wants.

The most important thing to understand about safe words is that they are not negotiable. A safe word is like an emergency ejector seat: If at any time your partner feels unsafe or uncomfortable, he or she can say the safeword, and then everything stops immediately. No one is allowed to criticize or question the use of a safe word because that is a jerk move and could make it harder for your partner to use the safe word next time she needs it. Having a safe word recognizes that your game is only happening because you both want it and are enjoying it.

As the dom, you need to make sure that your partner feels comfortable using the safe word if she needs to. But you should also be trying to make sure she never has to.

Read His Mind:

An important aspect of the dom's job is empathy. You may not associate empathy with the Big Bad Dom, but BDSM works best when the top can tell what the bottom is thinking. But what if you don't have ESP? The trick is to pay attention. Watch how your partner moves, listen to his breathing, feel how he responds to you, and you'll get a pretty good idea of his mindset. Watch how he reacts when you try out different moves. If you're planning to try a new trick that neither of you have done before, take it extra slow. If possible, you should try things out yourself before you inflict them on your partner. For example, if you're going to be using hot wax, test out how the wax feels on your own body before you go dripping it all over your partner. You can see how this can help you keep your games safe and fun— you're less likely to accidentally burn your partner if you know what you're working with!

You Make the Rules

THE MOVE

Now that you're versed on the responsibilities, it's time to get you cracking the (figurative) whip! One of the best ways to flex your authority is by issuing orders and setting rules. If your partner fails to follow directions, you get to decide what punishment to hand out. These commands and rules don't have to be all about sex—you're showing your partner that you're in charge, so your orders should emphasize that you're the boss. Your rules should be arbitrary—that's the point! The rules are only there so that you can enforce them, and so that your partner can submit to them.

MAKING IT HAPPEN

Just as with everything else in this book, there's no right or wrong way to do this. There's a huge range of ways that people act out this power play, and you don't have to wear a leash and call each other "slave" and "master" (unless you want to). Getting into your roles can be an adjustment, so take it slow like with the other moves. Here are some ideas to get you started:

Say my Name: Have your partner call you something sexy. You could go with the basic "Sir," or "Ma'am," or even "Master," but if that feels more silly than sexy, come up with something on your own. Submissives often refer to themselves in third person, which can get tricky if you're not used to it, so that might be a fun challenge to add to your play.

Fetch: Order your partner to get something for you. Whatever you want: a glass of water, a magazine, or that toy from across the room. You can think of this as a standard "because I said so" kind of command—whatever the exact reason for of the request, the real purpose is just to exercise your power.

Playing Dress Up: Tell your sub what to wear. This is fun just for sexy time, especially if you have some sexy lingerie or kinky costumes to bust out. Or have your partner wear something sexy just for you before they head out for the day: it could be their sexiest underoos, or special jewelry or accessory.

PUNISHMENT

THE MOVE

You've laid down the law, but it doesn't mean anything without a little enforcement. In fact, it is much better to think of your role as the dom to be enforcing, rather than punishing. When you're playing BDSM and your partner breaks a rule or disobeys orders, a "punishment" is useful to reinforce the dom's authority and the rules of the game. It can also give you a good chance to try some spanking techniques that you both enjoy in a "realistic" context.

Think about your punishment like the penalty in a drinking game. It's like when you miss a shot in beer pong and you have to chug—it's not personal, and it's not because the dom is angry with the sub for breaking the rules; it's just how you play the game. With that in mind, you should also remember that BDSM is *not* the time to work through real-life conflicts, and you should never punish your partner for real-world transgressions.

MAKING IT HAPPEN

How you hand out your punishments, and what kind of punishments you use is entirely up to you, so be creative! Your punishments don't have to be painful—in fact, unless you both enjoy a little pain with your pleasure, you can leave the belt at the door.

When you're playing around in the bedroom, it can be fun to issue sexy orders. You can have your partner touch themselves, or do something for you. You might want to think twice before choosing a sexytime staple as your punishment—do you really want to characterize a blow job as "punishment?" So make your "punishment" something new—you have a whole book of ideas here to choose from.

To really flex your dom muscles, you can assign punishments that benefit you—you are the boss, after all. Have your sub rub your feet, fix you a drink, maybe braid your hair or do your laundry. Think outside the box on this one.

"Oh then! the fiery touch of his fingers determines me, and my fears melting away before the glowing intolerable heat, my thighs disclose of themselves, and yield all liberty to his hand."

—John Cleland
Memoirs Of Fanny Hill

You can even make a punishment game with your partner by making a list of possible punishments beforehand, and numbering the list. Then when you need to punish your partner, have them roll a set of dice. Whatever number they land on is the punishment you use. If you don't have dice, you can write them on slips of paper and draw them from a hat. This works well if you two switch roles.

It's Your Scene

THE MOVE

In the kink world these pre-planned sexcapades are called "scenes." That term works so well because even if you're not wearing a costume, you are putting on a show. The end game is for you and your partner to have a good time, and the dom gets to make sure that happens—you're the director. For this you have to plan ahead. What kinds of props do you want to use? What toys or accessories? Are you going to tie your partner up or leave 'em loose? You can mix and match the moves in this book, and add in your own flourishes as you go.

MAKING IT HAPPEN

When you put on a scene, you get to control all the little details, and as you play with bondage, submission, and sensations, you get to control what your partner feels and experiences. How delicious—absolute power! Your partner's tied to the tracks, and what part will you play? Are you the dastardly villain, the courageous hero . . . or are you the train?

When preparing for a scene, think about how your partner will experience everything you have planned. Even if you're just planning a simple bedroom romp, you can help your sub get into the groove by making sure the room temperature is comfortable, clearing any clutter that could get in your way, and removing things that could distract your sub, like pictures, the alarm clock, or anything like that. Think through the whole plan, and make sure you have everything you need. When you're finally ready for your sub, suit up, and get ready to put on a show.

GIRL-ON-TOP POSITIONS

Think only guys can play on top? Think again. Guys can lie back and enjoy being submissive, too. Here are some girl-on-top positions to get you thinking about your next scene.

Classic Cowgirl: Ride him, girl! You know this position. It's one step up from missionary, with him lying on his back, and you straddling him. This position works well with most of the wrist binding techniques, or you can use the spread eagle to tie him down all together. From your perch, you can set the speed and rhythm of your movement: Keep it slow, and keep him from picking up the pace before you're ready. Make small circles with your hips, like a hula dancer, as you move up and down.

Reverse Cowgirl: This position is simple, but you can tweak it to come up with a ton of variations! To get in this position, have your partner lie down and straddle him, facing his feet. Bend your knees and arch your back to help him slide in. You can stay in that position and use your legs to ride your partner, or you can try straightening your legs and using your upper body to rock your hips back and forth.

Sexy Pretzel: I'm sure there's another name for this position, but I like to call it the sexy pretzel. First have your partner sit in the middle of the bed (not up against the headboard) with his legs out in front of him. Sit between his knees with your legs on either side of him. Scoot forward as you wrap your legs around his torso until you're in a good position to slide him into you. This position is great: It's close and intimate, sturdy and doesn't require too much flexibility, and gives you plenty of leverage to move, twist and thrust in any way you want.

Love Seat: Beds get all the recognition as the most common lusty locale, but the common kitchen chair is a great unsung sexy hero, especially in the world of girl-on-top. As I mentioned earlier, this position is a great option for when you want to tie him up, and it's very versatile. For a big soft chair or a couch, have your partner sit, then straddle him with a knee on either side of his legs. Arch your back and lean backwards (holding his shoulders if you need support) to get the full effect. This ends up being a kind of cross between cowgirl and the pretzel position where you're partly perched and partly entwined, which makes for a double-whammy of pleasure, since this position is ideal for stimulating your clitoris as well as the elusive G-spot.

On a hard chair, like a dining room or desk chair, you have even more options for positioning. You can sit facing your partner, with your legs on either side of the chair. If your chair is short enough (or you're tall enough) you can use your legs to lift yourself up and lower yourself down again. Rotate your hips, and rub up against your partner. If you've got him tied up, you can tease him by playing with your nipples, stroking his chest, or pulling his hair. You can also try this position facing away from your partner. If he's bound, you may have trouble getting into the right position, so you may want to try this together before you tie him up. It's a tad trickier, but if he's an ass man, he'll like the view.

ABOUT THE AUTHOR

Marisa Bennett is a former English major with a definite kinky side! Her hard limits are ice cream with nuts and skydiving. She lives with her husband in Minnesota.

"It's the soul's
   duty to be loyal
to its own desires.
   It must abandon itself to its
master passion."

—Rebecca West

RESOURCES FOR NAUGHTY PLAY

BOOKS

365 Sex Positions: A New Way Every Day for a Steamy, Erotic Year
By the Editors of Amorata Press, Photography by Allan Penn

A sex position for every day of the year, this book features step-by-step explanations and sultry photography to help you spice up your sex life. Reminiscent of the *Kama Sutra*, this book gives a modern, clear, and stylish approach to enhancing your playtime.

The Seductive Art of Japanese Bondage
By Midori, Photography by Craig Morey

Featuring tasteful photos and descriptions of shibari, a form of Japanese rope bondage, this book expresses the philosophy, history, and poetic side of bondage, appealing to beginners and experienced BDSM enthusiasts alike.

Two Knotty Boys Showing You the Ropes: A Step-by-Step, Illustrated Guide for Tying Sensual and Decorative Rope Bondage
By Two Knotty Boys, Photography by Larry Utley
This instructional guide to ropes and bondage has in depth descriptions, safety guides, and imagery of tying both practical and decorative knots for your sexy scenes.

The Modern Kama Sutra: An Intimate Guide to the Secrets of Erotic Pleasure
By Kamini Thomas and Kirk Thomas
A modern take on the *Kama Sutra*, this book provides how-to descriptions of 40 sex positions, practical advice, and photography for anyone ranging from the sex newbie and the coital connoisseur.

"Only passions, **great** passions, can elevate the soul to great things."

—Denis Diderot

*What are some of your secret fantasies you'd
like to be able to share with your partner?*

_____

_____

_____

_____

_____

_____

_____

_____

_____

_____

_____

_____

_____

_____

_____

_____

_____

_____

_____

_____

_____

_____

_____

_____

What's something that makes you feel sexy? Is it a particular item of clothing? Or devouring a certain kind of food?

Write about a particular time or place in your life when you felt daring or naughty. Did you follow through on your desires? If so, why or why not?

_____

_____

_____

_____

_____

_____

_____

_____

_____

_____

_____

_____

_____

_____

_____

_____

_____

_____

_____

_____

_____

_____

Have you read any books or blogs that have turned you on? Try reading them aloud to your partner and see what happens!

_____
_____
_____
_____
_____
_____
_____
_____
_____
_____
_____
_____
_____
_____
_____
_____
_____
_____
_____
_____
_____

*Write about a sexual goal you'd like to achieve
for yourself and your relationship.*

_____

_____

_____

_____

_____

_____

_____

_____

_____

_____

_____

_____

_____

_____

_____

_____

_____

_____

_____

_____

_____

_____

Write your own sexy tips and secrets here—and remember to refer back to them for ideas!

_____

_____

_____

_____

_____

_____

_____

_____

_____

_____

_____

_____

_____

_____

_____

_____

_____

_____

_____

_____

_____

_____

"There is no remedy
for love but to
love
more."

—Henry David Thoreau
The Journal of Henry David Thoreau
1837-1861

"There's always one who loves and one who lets himself be loved."

—W. Somerset Maugham
Of Human Bondage